Shift

Simple Guide to Helping Busy Ladies Think Differently and Get Their Bodies Back

Matt Fruci, ANutr, MSc, BSc

Shift

Printed by:
CreateSpace Independent Publishing Platform

Copyright © 2017, Matt Fruci, ANutr, MSc, BSc

Published in the United States of America

170704-00849.3

ISBN-13: 978-1979784498
ISBN-10: 1979784493

For more information on 90-Minute Books including finding out how you
can publish your own book, visit 90minutebooks.com or call (863) 318-0464

DISCLAIMER

While the author of this book has carried out extensive research and has thus attempted to make information as regards to his findings conveniently available through this medium; the writer and the distributor will not be held accountable for any harm resulting from the misinterpretation of any information contained therein. All information suggested are directly drawn from available data and may not be suitable for all circumstances and scenarios. It is therefore the duty of the user of this book to ensure that they are upholding all national and international laws as well as applying the information contained here to the situations that are best fitting for it

HERE'S WHAT'S INSIDE...

Introduction 1

Why Is It So Difficult For Busy Ladies To Lose
Weight And Keep It Off? 5

Shift! 8

The Six Principles To Think Differently And
Get Your Body Back 10

Principle #1
Control Circle 10

Principle #2
Creating More Time For You. Creating
Your Get To Do List 12

Principle #3
Decluttering Your Brain and Your
Kitchen To Lose Weight And Tone Up ... 25

Principle #4
How To Lose A Stone In 24 Hours 29

Principle #5
The Shift Audit 36

Principle #6
Break The Habit 38

This Works For Busy Ladies Regardless
Of What They've Tried Before 42

How Busy Ladies Can Make The Shift,
Tone Up, And Get Their Bodies Back
For Good 48

Bonus: Meal Ideas To Save You Time And Money And Get You Enjoying Your Food Again.................................... 50

Snack Ideas So You Don't Have To Hide The Wrappers... 53

Here's How To Think Differently And Get Your Body Back 60

*To my beautiful wife and daughter – my strong
support all the way through my intriguing journey*

-Matt Fruci

Introduction

"My head feels like mashed potato...
but should I use sweet potato or white potato?
Or both? Or carrot? Swede?
Sod it, pass me the ice cream"

-Matt Fruci

Why is it so difficult to lose weight and keep it off? I mean, just check out these statistics below:

50% of us have been on a diet in the last year with limited success.

Two-thirds would have regained more weight than we lost in the first place.

It's 2017, and we're still struggling to lose weight and keep it off. Isn't this crazy? I thought we had it figured out. Experts are telling you that fat is bad one minute, while in the next, sugar is bad and fat is good for you. It's irritating and frustrating. So I understand that this makes you think this way: "I tried to eat healthily but it turns out what I was doing was wrong, so I might as well just eat what I want"... and you give up.

It's a pain, this weight loss and toning up stuff. From what you've been told, it's time-consuming, confusing, and scary. You don't want to spend hours in an intimidating gym full of twenty-year-olds chucking weights around. You don't want to have to give up your carbs and prosecco and live off of chicken and broccoli for the rest of your life. And you want to enjoy meals out with friends and family.

I've been there. You see, all of these detoxes and diets, the 'blame sugar,' 'blame fat,' 'ditch gluten,' and 'count your sins' diets just remind me of the old, anorexic Matt. That's right, before doing my postgraduate research in nutrition, and becoming a Registered Nutritionist who would go on to help hundreds of ladies lose weight and ditch the 'good-bad' and 'all-or-nothing' dieting mentality, I battled with anorexia.

And I see these elements in all those fad diets people get told to do, leading them through this vicious cycle:

Diet starts Monday → Deprive yourself of the foods you love → Lose weight → Get stressed and tired → Binge → Feel like a failure → Binge a bit more → Put on more weight → Diet starts Monday → Repeat

But I'm here to tell you that it's not your fault. What if the diet itself simply wasn't fit for your lifestyle?

This is why I resonate with so many busy ladies. Because I had a poor relationship with food whilst growing up, I don't always eat perfectly. I am vulnerable to the odd binge on coconut chocolate if I don't arrange my environment to WIN. That is the reason why I have written this book: to make things super simple for you, so you don't have to rely on your willpower and can build a nutritional strategy that suits your lifestyle. No more of that comment, 'Oh, you're not on another diet' from the other half; no more eating separately or missing out on social events with loved ones. Just simple, powerful habits that, if used correctly, will give you more energy and help you think differently about dieting so you can take control of your comfort eating and get your body back for good.

You see, it doesn't matter about the latest diet tip that you get off Facebook or from your friend who's just lost 10 pounds in 10 days unless you've got your mindset in the right place. Because that will just set you up for failure. I mean, just by speaking with the ladies on my Body Transformation programmes and reading the gossip mags my wife picks up, it's no secret that you're bombarded with fad diets telling you to 'eat raw food only', 'only eat wholemeal foods', 'ditch the carbs', 'only eat organic'; all of these activities are full-time jobs in themselves! That is why I always say to the ladies I work with:

Can you see yourself doing this in 12 weeks, in six months? Even in 12 months' time? Because if you can't, are you setting up yourself for failure?

Just like undigested foods can make you feel sluggish and tired, undigested experiences (i.e. not learning from your mistakes) can leave you doing the same old diet and expecting different results. It's why I get people to think differently about their diets. We start with a focus on what you can control to empower you to put yourself first, and prioritise those items that are most important to you. When you ask someone, "How are you," they start moaning about things completely out of their control: weather, traffic, what others have said and done, etc. But you have no control over all these things. Despite this, we spend most of our time, energy and emotion in these areas, which drain our willpower and leave us compensating by making less-informed, irrational decisions, leading us towards comfort eating and acting irritable with loved ones. But what if you just focused on the areas you CAN control? What would be different?

Enjoy the book!

I hope this book empowers you to shift away from the 'good-bad,' 'all-or-nothing' dieting mindset towards a sustainable approach that you can stick to, so you can get your body back for good and—dare I say it—have a bit of fun in the process.

To Your Shift!

Matt Fruci

Why Is It So Difficult For Busy Ladies To Lose Weight And Keep It Off?

"If you can't see yourself doing this diet in 12 weeks, six months or a year, are you setting yourself up to fail?"

–Matt Fruci

Think about all the conflicting information that you get on social media from friends and family, such as 'ditch the carbs.' Or have you seen this one? You are supposed to only eat as a caveman would: no sugar, no carbohydrates—only eat meat, nuts and berries. These are the very same cavemen who were lucky to live to see 30 years old.

All of this conflicting information can be incredibly confusing. You're told to give up gluten and eat only raw foods, and that you must eat breakfast even if you're on the go and don't have time. So you scoff down something, grabbing anything on the go to boost your metabolism and stop you from going into fat storage mode (ever been told that one?), but all of these types of eating are almost full-time jobs in themselves. The time involved makes you less likely to stick to the programme, which is essentially the most important thing. If you can't see yourself doing the buying and prepping of all of these special meals in six months or 12 months, are you setting yourself up for failure?

One of the most common remarks I hear from members on my Body Transformation programmes is this: "I'm so sorry, Matt. I skipped breakfast today and I know that's bad." Often there is no reasoning behind this idea; it's just assumed that skipping breakfast is 'bad' because you're told that breakfast spikes your metabolism, and stops you going into 'fat storing mode' where your body apparently clings on to fat. I'm trying to imagine someone clinging on to their fat as I write this.

You see, if you're not enjoying the food at that time anyway and just scoffing anything down to spike your metabolism, could breakfast be making you fat?

I see busy ladies getting in their 6:00 a.m. breakfast before a busy day at work, whether or not they are hungry, only to be starving at 9:00 a.m. at their desk, where they just grab anything and everything anyway. Sometimes the solution can be to pack something and take it to work with you to eat when you are hungry, even if that means you don't eat until 11 am. Yes, even if you have your first meal at 11 am, this is still breakfast. After all, breakfast simply means 'breaking the fast'.

For other ladies I work with, having breakfast can help curb their hunger; it stops them snacking at mid-morning, and it's why there is no one-size-fits-all solution here. It's neither 'breakfast is good' or 'breakfast is bad', it's your overall intake and what you do on average. If having breakfast stops you thinking about food all morning, that's good. If you're not enjoying it, and you have breakfast at 6:00 a.m. or 7:00 a.m. before work, it's probably not doing you any good if you're not even hungry at that time and you're hungry later anyway.

The more you're told what and when to eat, the further you get away from listening to what your own body is telling you to do. Now, before you go 'listening to your body', just consider that this in itself could be pretty dangerous advice. Just by smelling the bacon sandwiches in your favourite coffee shop or being offered a £1 chocolate bar at the checkout in the supermarket can be enough to make you think you're hungry. It's why for some ladies, eating by the clock might actually work. It stops them from grabbing food between meals. My approach? Learn to listen to what works best for you versus trying to force yourself to eat one way because you saw a post on Facebook about it, and some stranger you don't know lost some weight following it.

Shift!

"The Best Diet In the World Is The One You Can Do"

–Matt Fruci

Before we get into some of the how-to methods, let's talk about the benefits of once and for all figuring out how to modify what you eat, so you no longer find yourself yo-yo-ing between starving and gorging yourself.

Imagine enjoying clothes shopping again, being in control of your relationship with food, and feeling like yourself again? Imagine being happy by looking at what you see in the mirror and feeling more confident about yourself? What would be different? Most ladies tell me, "Oh, I just want to lose weight," but really they want to fit into their favourite clothes and feel better. They want their belt notch to go down a hole, their bracelet to feel looser, to get their favourite dress back on, and to be happy about what they see in the mirror every day when getting dressed.

There are other benefits, such as increased confidence, having more energy, and being more productive, so you can come home from work and have the energy to have a social life and spend more time with your family doing the things you enjoy, of course.

It's important to get out of the mindset of thinking, "I'm too fat to do this," or that "identity habit" where you just say, "I'm the unfit one. I'm the fat one." It often stops you growing as a person and doing the things you need to do to get the things you say you want. If you're the unfit one, you live up to that reputation, and then you don't exercise. If you're the fat one, you don't make intelligent decisions about the foods you eat. I see ladies choosing to allow these deeply held beliefs to self-sabotage their progress.

If you can build a nutrition strategy that fits your lifestyle, so you're not thinking about diet and food all day, then you can focus on the things that really matter: family, friends, social life, enjoying your work, having fun, etc. When you have fun you feel good, right? So, let's talk about what you should be doing to get your body back and get you out into the world feeling great!

The Six Principles To Think Differently And Get Your Body Back

Principle #1
Control Circle

"Until you make the unconscious conscious, it will direct your life, and you will call it fate"

-Carl G Jung.

You see, when you ask someone how they are, they often start talking about things completely out of their control: the weather, traffic, what others have said and done. But all these things, you have no control over. Despite this, we spend most of our time, energy and emotion here, which drains our willpower and leaves us compensating by making less-informed, irrational decision, leading us to comfort eat and be irritable with loves ones. But what if we just focused on the areas we CAN control? What would be different?

To help you waste less time on the things that don't serve you so you can have more time to do what you enjoy, go to www.FruciFit.com/Circle to download your free Control Circle.

A task for you: Write down five things you've achieved that made you happy; next, write five things that happened that led to you feeling disappointed or let down. With the things that made you happy, were you 100% responsible for them? For the things that made you feel let down and disappointed, was it because you expected more from others? Shifted responsibility?

My point is that when you blame others by shifting the responsibility on to others, you become helpless. There is nothing you can do. When you choose to take full responsibility, you either win or you learn from every experience. If you win? Reflect on what worked well? If you learn? Well, this is where the breakthroughs are. What could you do differently? How could you improve? This will show you where you need to spend more of your energy.

Principle #2
Creating More Time For You.
Creating Your Get To Do List

"He who has their health has 1,000 dreams. He who doesn't has 1"

–Anon

The truth is that, if you don't make time for your health now, eventually you will have to make time for it. Something I'm adopting into my life is that if I want happy and healthy kids, I must be happy and healthy, right?

I think this quote sums it up nicely:

"He who has their health has 1,000 dreams. He who doesn't has 1"

Just as you do with your kids, I want to see my daughter grow up. I want to jump on the trampoline with her, take her swimming, take her away on trips, see her get married, lead by example, etc. After all, memories are what you remember most. But to do this, you must look after YOU. In this first section, I will show you three super simple ways to help you do this.

Why?

Because not taking care of you will eventually lead to poor management of stress, fatigue, and overwhelm. What do I mean?

Accumulated stress will escalate tiredness which results in less prefrontal cortex activation in your brain (which helps you make more intelligent, better-informed decisions about what you do and eat). The result is poor dietary decisions and being irritable around your loved ones. I've been there, too. Having little patience with my daughter and being snappy with my wife, just because I didn't look after me. The result? Comfort eating.

Step 1: Plan Your Family's Meals a Week In Advance to Save Time and Money.

Research has shown that (on average) a family rotates through 14 different meals. So, what if you could batch cook that spaghetti Bolognese or chilli con carne? Perhaps have Monday's spaghetti bowl, Wednesday's chilli and Friday's spaghetti bowl all ready to go for the next month in your freezer?

I've given you a blank Food Planning Template you can use to help you get organised. Go to www.FruciFit.com/diary to download your Food Planning template.

This is why you should do it:

- You can cook several weeks' worth of meals in one go, get back your 'ME' time, and have more time do other things you want to do (like spending time with your friends and family)

- You don't need to waste time every day, nipping out to the shops to grab 'whatever' for tea, as it will be done for you. Did you know the average supermarket trip takes 41 minutes? Did you also know that supermarkets place items they want you to buy at eye level and at the end of an aisle? Can you imagine spending less time wondering around a supermarket and more time with your loved ones?
- You would have planned your meals and snacks, so you never have to go shopping hungry (or h-angry, as my wife calls it). Research shows that hungry shoppers choose foods higher in calories and opt for the "SEE-food diet" (you grab everything you see).
- You'll have a shopping list, so you won't waste money on stuff you don't need.
- You'll be cooking less, which will dramatically reduce your electricity bills.

On the next page is a sample Food Planner. Go to www.FruciFit.com/diary to download your Food Planning template.

	Monday	Tuesday	Wednesday	Thursday	Friday	Saturday	Sunday
Breakfast							
Snack							
Lunch							
Snack							
Dinner							
Water	1 2 3 4 5 6 7 8	1 2 3 4 5 6 7 8	1 2 3 4 5 6 7 8	1 2 3 4 5 6 7 8	1 2 3 4 5 6 7 8	1 2 3 4 5 6 7 8	1 2 3 4 5 6 7 8

Fuci Fit

15

I see so many busy ladies blaming their 'willpower' for not sticking to it 100%. So I'm here to show you my philosophy, one that works:

When should I complete the planner?

When you have between 10 to 20 minutes. Many members of my Body Transformation programme do this on a Sunday and involve the family. One member of my Body Transformation programme does it while she waits for her kid to finish swimming. Put the time that suits you in your diary so you do it. If you can't tell me where your time has gone, you will always be time poor. Prioritise your day or someone else will prioritise it for you. Don't forget to also diarise a time to actually get the shopping you need.

I couldn't stick to it. I'm a failure.

So you make a plan, but you don't stick to it. Maybe you had some extra work, your other half was busier than normal, or things just didn't go 100% to plan. So you opted for that quick and easy Chinese takeaway.

Now, if I had a Chinese takeaway for every time I heard that, I suppose I would have... a million Chinese takeaways (which is a scary thought)...

This is the real question: what plan ever goes 100% to plan?

Half-assed is better than no-assed.

Ask yourself. If you believe that eating a Chinese takeaway will make you fat, do you think it will? My opinion? It will if you believe it will. Because what happens when you believe this Chinese buffet or takeaway was BAD? You choose to drift away from what works. You see, one Chinese takeaway probably won't hurt. Three Chinese takeaways, a multipack of crisps, and half a cheesecake— probably will. So, let me ask you this: Is it the Chinese Takeaway that's the problem or is it your belief that having a Chinese Takeaway means you've failed (which is what they tell you in most of the cookie-cutter diet plans you see in the magazines and Slimming Clubs)?

Step 2: Download Your Shift Confidence Worksheet By Going To www.FruciFit.com/Confidence

Shift Confidence	Specific Action	Further Progression	Why	Win
Monday 1				
2				
3				

This helps you to count your wins and add them up every week…

Imagine if you wrote down 3 things you did well every, single day? That's 21 wins a week and 84 wins a month. What a year that could be (I'll let you do the math). All of which would suggest you're not doing too badly, after all.

How to use your Confidence Shift:

Start each day by writing down three things you did well on the previous day. This is a way for you to appreciate a 'win' for the day before. Write why this is a 'win' and how you can make further progress with this.

- Win = planning your family meals for the week.
- Why = shopping list done, saved money, one less thing to worry about, the family knows what's for dinner, less buying on the go.
- Further progress and action = plan one week of food ahead each Sunday at 8am before the family are up.

Whatever time suits you, put it in your diary right now, so it becomes REAL.

Now let me ask you this: What if you slowed down and just accepted that the Chinese takeaway happened? Perhaps planned to alter your food intake a little bit tomorrow? Accepted that 80% is 'good enough' and better than yesterday? Moved away from the 'good/bad,' 'all-

or-nothing' mentality, and just accepted that nothing is perfect? Would the gap, between where you are right now and where you want to be, get any smaller?

Why is this powerful? Because doing this exact task – which I call Shift Confidence – gives you the confidence to have the courage to continue and shift away from that vicious yo-yo dieting cycle we talked about earlier. It helps you stay calm when you'd usually lose your $#*!.

And this is the difference between starting and stopping all of the time and getting in the best body shape of your life (regardless of your age). That is, your ability to keep going. And in my opinion, this comes from protecting your confidence. Showing an appreciation of the results that you are achieving. No matter how small. After all, your brain is not designed to make you feel good. It's designed to look for stress in your life. That's how we've survived this long. So, it's our responsibility to remind ourselves of our wins every, single day. After all, no one else will. So, don't be shy. Give yourself a pat on the back 3 times a day.

Step 3: Be More Selfish. Your Family and Friends Will Thank You for It

I remember this cold and wet evening. I had finished late from work, hungry (or 'H-angry', as my wife calls me), tired, and stressed. My wife came in while I was washing up and put two dirty tumblers on the side. Visibly irritated, I turned to her and moaned: "Could you not have just used the same glass?"

Do you see what happened there? Not looking after ME meant I was short and snappy with the love of my life; the most important person in my life. And the same happens when I'm with my daughter. If I haven't looked after *me*, my patience is tested, and I'm not great to be around. Not only this, what do you turn to when you feel like this to make you feel better? Yep, that delicious, melt-in-the-mouth creamy, fudge brownie ice cream.

This is why I will tell you to be more selfish. Because when you and I find ourselves being snappy and more irritable with loved ones, it's usually because we haven't put ourselves first. Now, you're probably thinking that this sounds a bit negative. After all, one of the Brownie club promises is to think of others first. But, if the queen is empty, how can she look after her people?

So I will show you how, in just three minutes, you COULD become less irritable with your family, friends and even your boss; you could become more fun to be around, and get on your way to fitting into your favourite, more fashionable clothes. How about if I were to tell you to take a pill that did all these things:

- Boosted your energy levels so you could be more productive, have more fun, and do more of the things you want to do

- Made you less irritable with your kids and your other half
- Helped reduce your hunger so you could gain control of your food cravings, and make better-informed, more intelligent food choices
- Boosted your immune system so you could prevent and overcome colds and illnesses rapidly
- Helped to ease achy joints and improve your bone health
- Meant you were less out of breath when climbing the stairs and doing everyday tasks so you could be your best self
- Improved your quality of sleep so you could wake up feeling refreshed and full of energy
- Inspired your friends, family, and kids to be fit, strong, and healthy.

Would you take it? Every day, right? Well, this 'pill' is exercise. And right now, I know what you're thinking:

- 'I don't have time to exercise.'
- 'Exercise is boring.'
- 'I don't have a gym membership.'
- 'The slimming clubs never told me how to exercise to tone up in quick, fun, and simple way'

But I'm here to tell you that even three minutes can make a huge difference; this is the way many ladies on my body transformation programmes start their journey.

Also, you can do it at home, before any of your family are up, just like the members on my body transformation programmes do. I mean, if you hit snooze on your alarm clock for 10 minutes every day of the year, that's 3650 minutes wasted. All I'm asking you to do is commit to 3 minutes.

Now, pick something you enjoy and do it tomorrow. Put it in your diary now.

DO NOT PUT IT OFF. Otherwise, you won't do it.

Now, maybe I lied a little bit. Because bringing in three minutes of exercise a day ALONE probably won't get you back your body for good.

But this is where the magic happens. Maybe you lose one pound in the first week. You gain a bit of confidence. Maybe you decide to do an extra minute this week? You start to feel better about yourself. You think clearly. You have more energy. You're starting to feel fit, have more energy and are less reliant on coffee to get you through the day. Then you lose another few pounds... Decide to make a few changes to your diet. Drink more water. Leave a fruit bowl out on the side. Leave prepared veggies in the fridge to make them easy to grab. Your family and friends then start commenting on how great you look, even asking you how you've done it.

Do you get where I'm going with this? The best thing you can do is START. You only get results for DONE. You can say 'it won't work for me' or 'I'm different.' But ask yourself, how do you know this? Are you psychic? If so, please forward the lottery numbers for this Saturday to matt@frucifit.com, Mystic Meg. Joking apart, the only sure way this will NOT work for you is if you say, 'I can't do it, it won't work for me.'

I get it. It's so simple that you probably won't do it. But here's the thing—that shiny, silver bullet does not exist. Get started NOW and your only regret will be that you didn't start earlier.

Principle #3
Decluttering Your Brain and Your Kitchen To Lose Weight And Tone Up

I remember a while back, my wife came home and started on one of those 'health kicks.' You know, where you get loads of 'natural' foods that promise to give you superpowers that Batman could only dream of! Nuts, seeds, wholemeal bread, dark chocolate, goji berries, coconut, you name it—all good stuff which is supposed to be eaten under the guidance of a nutritional strategy that considers your exercise habits, lifestyle, sleep, and necessary fat loss. But what happened when my wife put the goji berries in a bowl on the side mixed with nuts and seeds? Every time I walked past them, I'd find myself taking a handful, whether I was hungry or not. Whether I had just finished my Sunday roast or not.

You see, you eat with your eyes, not your stomach. In fact, did you know that you eat 92% of what you serve on your plate?

So, these eight bulletproof tips will help you take control of your 'demons' that make you finish the pack of sour cream and onion crisps that your family keep bringing into the house, so you can stop blaming your willpower and get your body back for good.

(These tips are courtesy of the researchers at Cornell University... their work is AMAZING.)

1. **Use small crockery** - This can reduce your food intake by 22%. (This tip alone could help you lose 40 pounds in a year...talk about 'dieting' without going on a 'diet'.)

2. **Sit down to eat** - This will help you eat less. How much do you mindlessly eat while on-the-go?

3. **Tidy up** – In a messy kitchen with paper/books left out, the toaster on the side, dishes in the sink ('Whose turn was it to load the dishwasher?'), you are likely to eat twice as much compared with someone whose kitchen was tidy. In the Cornell study, women ate 53 more calories from...cookies when their kitchen was messy!

4. **'Don't use your counter as a buffet'** - Women who left out cereal on their kitchen counters were 20 pounds heavier than those who didn't. Those who displayed fizzy drinks weighed 26 pounds more. Those who had a fruit bowl weighed 13 pounds less.

5. **Use snack blockers** – This can help you become more mindful about the amount you are eating. For example, choosing fruits you have to peel or prepare, like

oranges, will slow you down and potentially stop you from overeating.

6. **Have a snack cupboard** – You make over 200 decisions about food every single day. How much should you eat? When should you eat it? Is this too much? Am I hungry? Should I eat now as I'm going out? Should I use a tablespoon? A teaspoon? Plate? Bowl? This drains your willpower quite enough, right? My advice is to have a snack cupboard. Put every available snack, like crisps and chocolate, into ONE cupboard. Why? If you WANT a snack, you will now have to make a rational, conscious decision to open that ONE cupboard, rather than opening a cupboard to get out the rice only to be tempted by chocolate biscuits (which means you can stop blaming the kids and hubby)

7. **Have a plan** – Yes, planning again! Use the meal planner to compile your shopping list. Research shows that you will buy lower calorie foods and be less tempted by checkout promotions, which will save you time and money!

8. **Have six high-protein snacks handy** – Protein helps keep you more full for a longer amount of time. These snacks could be Greek yoghurts, cooked chicken leftovers (perhaps from your roast

chicken), smoked salmon, tinned tuna, eggs, whey protein powder, ham, or even cheese. Make it easy for yourself to grab something quick that is not full of sugar, and out of a packet, so you can get away from those sugar highs and lows!

If you don't set up your environment to win, by default you're setting yourself up for failure. Just like I recently did. You see, every time I go the hygienist, they tell me to floss. I think, 'Right, I'm going to do it.' I buy the floss, and do it consistently for a few weeks. The floss runs out, and then I forget about it. Why? All because it wasn't next to my toothbrush. You see, had it been there, I would have done it. Bet you didn't think you could learn so much from some dental floss, right?

Principle #4
How To Lose A Stone In 24 Hours

Don't eat, don't drink, and jump around in a sauna. My point is that weighing scales can be as truthful as Pinocchio at times, and this has been the case for many members of my Body Transformation programmes. You feel like you're doing everything right: drinking water, eating fruit and veggies, and walking more, yet you still gained two pounds this week. And what happens afterward?

You adopt the 'F it' mindset... Eat the rest of the chocolate biscuits, and even pinch the ones in your kid's 'treat cupboard' (hoping they forgot about those chocolate buttons), all because of the number on the scales. The truth is—especially when starting out—what you do is MORE important than the outcome. You see, if you focus so much on the scales, you forget about the things you are doing (or NOT doing, in some instances). Ultimately, how you look and feel in 90 days (or six to twelve months from now), is a direct result of your daily, consistent habits—not the number on the scales two weeks into a new diet. Even though most new members on my Body Transformation programme would say something like this, "I want to lose weight and tone up," what they mean is this: "I want my clothes to fit better, and I want to feel more confident in my skin."

This is exactly why I'm going to show you the nine reasons why the scale might go up as you start dieting. So you can remain calm, focus on changing your body shape, fit your clothes better and – dare I say it - ENJOY the process of ditching your love handles and getting your body back – stress-free!

You've started eating more fruit and vegetables

Fibre is hard for your body to break down. It can make you gassy and bloated; this also means you hold more water. Consider that you're probably going to eat different amounts of fibre each day – which can impact your weight!

The good news? Over time, your body will probably get better at handling your increased fibre intake; you'll feel more full and stop craving more sugary, high-fat snacks and foods which could help you lose FAT, so you fit your clothes better!

You've started drinking more fluids

Yep, another positive habit could make you put on more weight, at least in the short term. It could be from tea, coffee, water, squash, or even Diet Coke. I mean, you exercise one day and maybe not the next. You may sweat a lot one day (weather/exercise) and not so much the next. The good news? Over time, your body will better regulate this increased fluid intake, you'll feel more full and satisfied, and stop mistaking thirst for hunger.

You eat more salt one day compared to another

Perhaps you started preparing your meals. Maybe you've started keeping higher protein snacks in the fridge, like smoked salmon, turkey ham, eggs, cheese, and natural yoghurt. Maybe you've been making some wraps with some cold meats on-the-go.

If you have been trying to increase your protein intake (which helps you feel more full and reach that more toned, leaner look), by doing so, you may have increased your salt intake – making you hold more water and increasing your weight!

Alternatively, changes could be due to something as simple as swapping supermarket rotisserie chicken one day for a home-roasted chicken on the next. The salt levels may be completely different in each instance. Perhaps you ate out at a restaurant where they probably don't care about the salt intake.

You ate higher carbs than normal today or a few days prior

For every gram of carbohydrates stored in your body, you pull about three or four grams of water into your muscles, which can mean you have gained water weight! This is NOT body fat.

Sleep

Some members of my Body Transformation programme will report LIGHTER body weights on the weekends. Why? Because they can sleep in (a bit) more, unless I'm knocking on their door at 7:15 a.m. as the wakeup call. So, consider that if you're in bed for a bit longer during the night, you may get up a few more times in the night and urinate more than normal (i.e. get rid of more water). If during the week, you only get five or six hours of sleep at night, the time between your last meal on the day before and your weigh-in will be shorter. This means your body may still be digesting the food, and having more food in your gut will mean that you weigh more.

You weren't consistent with time and day

Did you weigh yourself at the same time? Did you go to the bathroom before weighing yourself in the morning? Same underwear/ pyjamas?

You've started a new exercise programme

This is new for your muscles and is actually a stress for your body. But when you rest, the magic happens: your body repairs the muscles (you may feel a little bit achy at the start). Now, this process burns calories and will help you LOSE FAT!!! Yet...This 'magic process' AKA muscle recovery may mean that you increase your body weight (at least in the short term). Why? Because you're holding more water in the muscle to help your body REPAIR! Which is a bit like what your immune system does when you're struggling with hay fever. On top of this, if you're doing toning up exercises, you are sending a message to your body to shape up and get lean. This 'lean up' process means you are holding on to lean muscle, which actually weighs more than fat, so even though you could be fitting your clothes better and your waistline is shrinking, the scales may not reflect this.

You haven't done what you said you would do

This one HURTS. It makes you reflect on what YOU have (or have not) done. Have you done the work? Have you done what you said you would do? Do you need more support and accountability from like-minded ladies so you don't lose motivation?

Menstrual cycle

You know better than me about this one. That pre-menstrual phase 'bloat' can leave you holding more water (and craving carbs).

To sum up: For these nine reasons, your scales may not be dancing to the tune in your head. Remember, the scale is NOT your dictator or your boss—it's just one of many.

Here's what I suggest to monitor your progress:

- Progress pictures (for your reference, even if you scroll back through your Facebook photos)

- How you feel (energy wise, bloating, exercise habits)
- How you feel when you look in the mirror (how confident do you feel?)
- How you fit your clothes
- Have you done what you said you would do (workouts, monitored food intake, done something fun for you to help you feel good about yourself and manage stress, got to bed on time)?

These are the best tools you have, which is exactly what we do in my Body Transformation programme. After all, as a member on my Body Transformation Programme said: "Who cares how much I weigh if I feel confident on the beach in my bikini?"

I've learned through coaching many ladies that if you make small, manageable improvements on your journey, you'll learn exactly what your body needs to do to lose FAT (not just weight), so you can feel more confident in your favourite clothes again.

At times, your journey will be tough. You'll have days where you questions whether it's working. You might even want to self-sabotage all of your results I've been there many times, too (those times when I've stepped on the scales, phoned up the Specs shop, and asked for a full refund...). But my advice to you is to slow down and give yourself a chance to RESPOND to the situation. Will binging or giving up take you any closer to where you say you want to be with your feelings and body shape?

Measure your progress using what are known as PROCESS goals.

These could include a few or many activities:

- Increasing your steps.
- Trying a new, fun type of exercise.
- Increasing your fruit, veg and water intake, etc.
- Doing something fun for you (as how you do you feel and who do you become when you have fun?)

Principle #5
The Shift Audit

'I know that already!'. If I had a penny for every time I heard that one…well, you can best imagine. In my opinion, knowing and not DOING is as good as not knowing, which is why I put together this super simple Shift Audit. I'm giving you seven strategies you can add straight into your busy routine TODAY. Strategies that will help you tone up without draining your willpower or stressing you out.

So, what I need you to do is tick off each task you do every…single…day. Score yourself out of seven each week and have a little look in the mirror along the way. Remember, consistency TRUMPS perfection. And DOING crushes THINKING, but only 110% of the time. Go to www.FruciFit.com/Audit to download and print your audit.

The shift Audit

♥ **DAY:**

♥ **MY 7 KEYS FOR TODAY**
(1 POINT FOR EACH KEY YOU DO)

🍷 #1 I sat down to eat my food

🍷 #2 I ate my food from crockery (instead of out the packet)

🍷 #3 I drank a glass of water before each meal

🍷 #4 I waited 20 minutes before going for seconds

🍷 #5 I did 10,000 steps & tried a 3 minute workout

🍷 #6 I acknowledged that being 'full' and 'having enough' are different

🍷 #7 I ate 5 DIFFERENT fruit & vegetables

OVERALL SCORE: / 7

WWW.FRUCIFIT.COM

37

Principle #6
Break The Habit

So, you've set yourself this new goal of how you want to look and feel.

This new vision of how many pounds you're going to lose and the shops you're going to buy your new, more fashionable clothes from; let's say you decide on 24 pounds lost in 12 weeks, and you want to be able to do ten push-ups.

So, Monday comes around. You're motivated—as excited as little kids on Christmas Eve, or even you when eating Santa's mince pie and half of Rudolf's carrot. But Wednesday comes. And life just takes over. There are just too many obstacles. Your washing is piling up, work is taking more of your precious time than ever, your other half is working late, you're shattered, and all you want is a bit of 'me' time. So you just give up on all of this healthy living stuff.

But I'm here to tell you that it's not your fault. That this 'bad' habit of giving up when life gets hard is simply because of these 'all or nothing' diet fads they tell you to do. To break this 'bad' habit, you simply need to have a BREAKthrough. And these breakthroughs will only come from your obstacles. Imagine if you used your energy to create a simple strategy to overcome every obstacle you ever had? That took away any 'barriers' or instinct habits that would usually stop you doing what you know you should be doing to get the things you say you want?

Let's do a few examples:

Obstacle 1: I won't have time to workout today because [insert reason here].

> **Strategy 1**: I'll start off with a three-minute workout first thing in the morning so nothing can get in the way.

Obstacle 2: I won't have time to get the ingredients I need for the dinners.

> **Strategy 2:** I'm going to do my shopping on a Monday and take my shopping list. I'll then cook in bulk.

But I get it. It's not your fault. You have the airbrushed magazines making you feel guilty for not dedicating your life to the gym and exercising to get a flat tummy. The greedy supplement companies telling you that you have to use their 'fat burning' drinks to lose weight. The commercial gyms not giving you the support and accountability you need. The slimming clubs promoting their yoyo dieting stuff. Which all makes this toning up stuff hard, slow and frustrating.

So, now it's your turn.

You can download a free copy of 'The Shift Habit Breaker' at www.FruciFit.com/HabitBreaker

Shift Habit Breaker

"The Obstacles Lead You to The Outcome"	
Name	
Today's Date	
Target Date & Goal	

	A) Obstacles	B) Strategies
1		
2		
3		
4		
5		
6		
7		
8		

This Works For Busy Ladies Regardless Of What They've Tried Before

Fat Loss Mastery Body Transformation Member, Cassie:

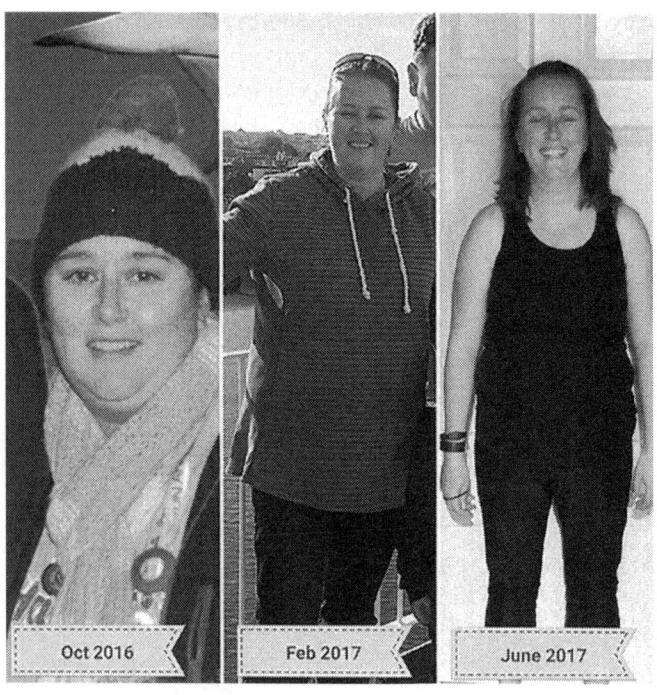

Oct 2016 · Feb 2017 · June 2017

"I have spent the last year feeling very unwell and gaining lots of weight as a result. I know I didn't have control over my body—that was what was so scary. I reached a point where I determined within

me that enough was enough. I wanted to be able to get on the floor and play with my family again, but I couldn't.

Starting out with Matt was the best thing I have ever done. He modified the exercises to work within my limitations. The food is easy, quick and the family time is not compromised because of this. We have enough opportunity to plan with lots of different choices; this plan is certainly helping us manage one of the stresses that are encountered by people like me who lead busy lives."

At the time she wrote this, Cassie has lost nearly four stone (and her other half has lost nearly two stone). She is having more fun than ever with her kids, from getting stuck in with them on the trampoline, to taking them swimming. The best part? Cassie has thrown away her size 20 clothes and is now fitting into size 12!

Well done, Cassie!

Body Transformation member, Julie:

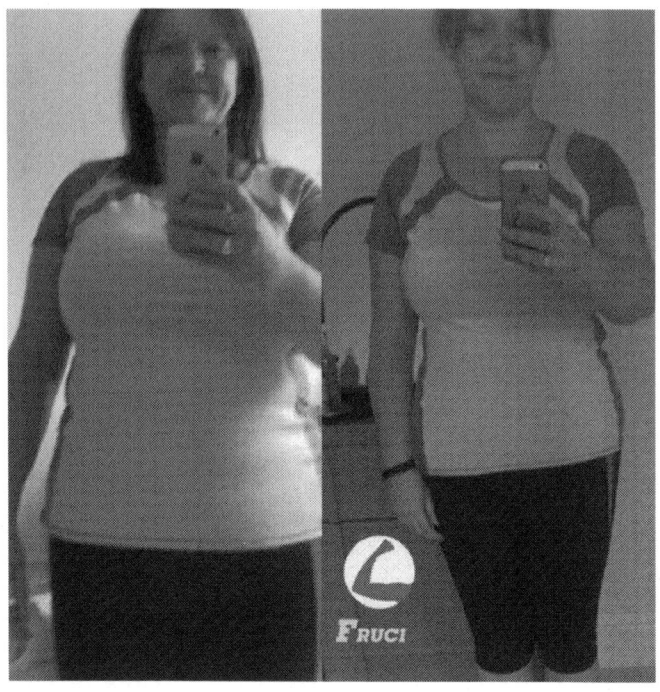

"I have tried so many diets in the past which resulted in very slow weight loss and then me getting disheartened and putting it all back on and more. Having recently changed jobs and able to commit more time to getting myself back to fitness and feeling good about the way I look I decided to try Matt's programme and I haven't looked back.

He has a simple approach to food. No gimmicks, just simple guidance, and weekly feedback if things need tweaking to get results. And the early morning fitness sessions are fun- and I'm not a morning person! But they set me up nicely for the day, giving me more motivation and inspiration to keep up with the diet and fitness programme throughout the week.

Matt gives great feedback and advice and keeps my motivation levels high each week. He encourages me to push myself more than I ever would myself.

I'm 7 weeks in and I've lost 10cm from my waist and friends have started to comment on how well I look. I have been surprised at how much extra energy I have despite doing considerably more activity each day, and my clothes are fitting better already If you are keen to make a difference to your health and fitness I would 100% recommend that you sign up to work with Matt."

Fat Loss Mastery Body Transformation Member Julie:

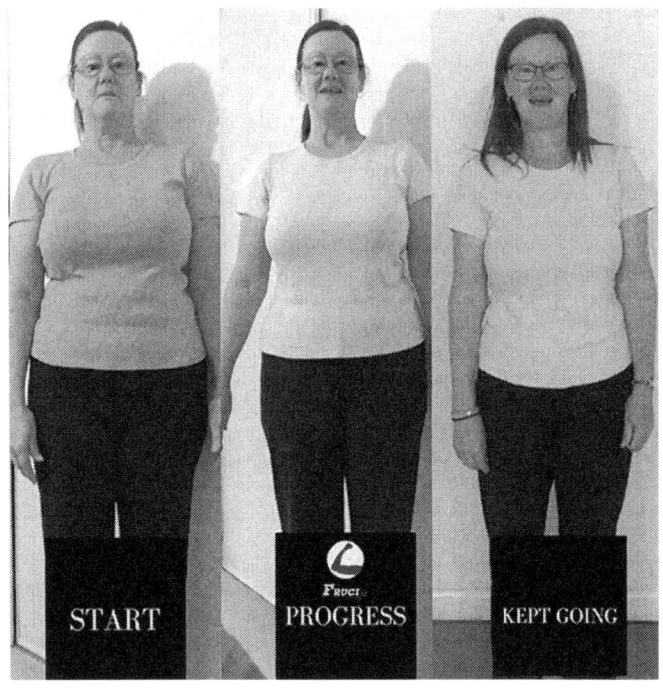

START PROGRESS KEPT GOING

"When I first started with Matt I felt disheartened with my body shape and never achieving my goal. I was fed up with going around in circles with diet and exercise and always landing back at square one. I was afraid of committing to something new in case I didn't succeed; however, those thoughts were quickly diminished once I met Matt.

Matt offers the whole package, a host of nutritious meals and exercise, and he helps you learn how to make better food choices. The biggest gain for me is knowing that I do not have to deprive myself of the things I love - and with that in mind, I know I will succeed. My attitude towards food has changed. I no longer crave what I can't have, but I am learning to moderate what I eat whilst knowing that my body is getting what it needs. I am just a few weeks into my programme, but I have already lost almost half a stone and 2.5 inches off my waist. My body is feeling more toned, and I feel positive about what the future will bring. If you are considering joining Matt, don't delay, do it now, and you won't look back."

How Busy Ladies Can Make The Shift, Tone Up, And Get Their Bodies Back For Good

Look. I know how it is. You've seen promises like this before. And maybe you're wondering, "is this really all that it's cracked up to be?" The answer is ... NO. **It's Even Better.**

Here's why: This isn't some "give up [insert food you love] here" diet where you're left overwhelmed, end up giving up and blaming your willpower and motivation.

I mean, you're already motivated! Otherwise, you wouldn't be reading this! **Here's Exactly What We'll Be Doing.**

You'll be shown a variety of fun, simple, and super quick toning up exercises throughout my Body Transformation programme to target your tummy fat, so you can get back into your favourite, more fashionable slimmer clothes (That's right, the best days are ahead of you!).

You get a step-by-step plan tailored and adapted for you and your lifestyle to guarantee that you stay on track and stick to it even on your worst day, no matter what life throws at you, be it the birthday cake day at work, lattes and cream teas with the ladies, the never-ending domestic admin, or the subtle and bubbly charms of prosecco.

You'll get support using the Fruci Fit Accountability System and gain access to **a** private supportive group of positive like-minded ladies so you don't lose motivation or feel alone like you would in a commercial gym.

Plus, you can gain access to the Fruci Fit Tone Up Kickstart App, so you no longer have to stress about knowing what to do for dinner or how to workout to slim down and tone up your tummy.

Your FREE personal 1-to-1 coaching session with me will help you ditch the yoyo dieting stuff they teach you at slimming clubs so you can build a sustainable diet that fits your lifestyle, tone up, get your body back for good, and – dare I say it – have more fun doing it.

Visit **www.FruciFit.com** and get started on making your Shift!

Bonus: Meal Ideas To Save You Time And Money And Get You Enjoying Your Food Again

Greek Turkey Burgers (Serves 4)

Shopping & Ingredients List:

- 500g Turkey Mince
- 150g Feta, crumbled
- 100g Green Olives, chopped
- 4 Spring Onions, chopped
- 1 tbsp dried Oregano
- Black Pepper, to own taste
- 2 tsp Olive Oil, for greasing

Method

1. Preheat grill to a medium-high heat. Can also use a bbq.

2. In a large bowl, combine turkey, feta cheese, olives, oregano & pepper. Mix together, form into patties.

3. Lightly oil the cooking grate or rack. Place patties on rack. Cook for 10 to 12 minutes, turning halfway through.

Nutritional info per serving

Protein	33.2g
Carbs	4.2g
Fat	15.2g
Energy	287Kcal

Chicken Fajitas (Serves 4)

Shopping & Ingredients List:

- 2 large Chicken Breasts, sliced
- 1 Red Pepper, deseeded & sliced
- 1 Red Onion, finely sliced
- bag of Mixed Salad
- 4 tbsp Fajita Seasoning
- 3 tbsp Olive Oil
- 4 Tortilla Wraps

Method

1. In a large wok heat olive oil & add the peppers, onion, chicken & seasoning

2. Cook over medium flame for 15 minutes, stirring frequently.

3. Spoon mixture into tortilla wraps.

4. Add some green salad. Roll the wrap up & serve while still warm.

Nutritional info per serving

Protein	**16g**
Carbs	**25g**
Fat	**4.2g**
Energy	**292Kcal**

Slow Cooker 'meals done for the week' Chilli Pork (Serves 12)

Shopping & Ingredients List:

- 5kg bone-in Pork Shoulder
- 2 x 400g tin Tomatoes (optional with Chilli)
- 1 Onion, chopped

Method

1. Place joint in slow-cooker. Top with onion & tinned tomatoes.

2. Cook on LOW for 10 hours. Remove from cooker & shred.

3. Serve with vegetables, salads, in lunch boxes. Great for producing several meals from one slow cooker.

Nutritional info per serving

Protein	69.7g
Carbs	2.9g
Fat	10.6g
Energy	387Kcal

Snack Ideas So You Don't Have To Hide The Wrappers

Pumpkin Pie Squares (Serves 9)

Shopping & Ingredients List:

- 10 pitted Dates, chopped
- 360g Oat Flour
- 2 tsp Pumpkin Pie spice (or 1 tsp cinnamon, ½ tsp ginger and ½ tsp ground nutmeg)
- 1 tsp Vanilla Extract
- 115ml Almond Milk

Method

1. Soak dates in 170ml water for 20 minutes. Lightly grease a 8"x 8" (20x20cm) baking tin and preheat oven to 190c (170 fan), 375f, gas mark 5.

2. Mix oat flour with pumpkin spice. Add soaked dates, water, vanilla extract, almond milk & blend until smooth.

3. Scrape batter into baking tin. Cook for 25 mins. Let cool for 10 mins before cutting & serving.

Nutritional info per serving

Protein	**7.5g**
Carbs	**46.3g**
Fat	**3.2g**
Energy	**245Kcal**

Super Filling Bean Brownies (Serves 3..but it could serve 6)

Shopping & Ingredients List:

- 240 g (1 tin) of drained red kidney beans (yes, you read that right...don't knock it until you try it)
- 80 ml of unsweetened almond milk
- 30 g of Gram flour (Chickpea flour...any will do but this is gluten-free)
- 15 g coconut flour
- 1 scoop of flavoured whey protein powder (I use cookies and cream flavour but any will do. You can substitute this for vanilla extract)
- 5 g cocoa powder
- 5 g sodium bicarbonate or baking powder
- A dash of cinnamon
- 1 tsp apple cider vinegar
- 1 egg
- 30 g quark or low fat soft cheese

Method

1. Blend all ingredients (apart from the toppings) in a blender and pour the mixture into a 'bread' tin sprayed with 1 kcal fry spray. Optional: Top with the chopped hazelnuts and chocolate

2. Place in the over for 20 mins or until you get a 'clean knife' at 180C

3. Leave to cool and serve!

Nutritional info per serving

Protein   **20 g**
Carbs   **26g**
Fat   **13g**
Energy   **300Kcal**

For a video showing you how to make this, go here: **www.frucifit.com/resist-cakes-starbucks/**

Kickstart Banana Bread (Serves 10)

Shopping & Ingredients List:

- 140g Wholemeal Flour
- 100g Self-Raising Flour
- 1 tsp Bicarbonate of Soda
- 1 tsp Baking Powder
- 300g mashed Ripe Bananas
- 4 tbsp Runny Honey
- 150ml 0% Greek Yogurt
- 3 Eggs, beaten
- 1 tsp Butter, melted

Method

1. Heat oven to 160c (140 fan), 325f, gas 3. Grease with melted butter & line a 2lb loaf tin with baking parchment (allow it to come 2cm above top of tin).

2. Mix the flours, bicarb, baking powder in a large bowl.

3. Mix the bananas, honey, eggs & yogurt. Quickly stir into dry ingredients, then gently scrape into the tin.

4. Bake for 1 hr 10 mins-1 hr 15 mins or until a skewer comes out clean.

5. Cool in tin on a wire rack. Eat warm or at room temperature.

Nutritional info per serving

Protein	**6g**
Carbs	**24g**
Fat	**2g**
Energy	**138Kcal**

<u>Strawberry Coconut Balls (Serves 7)</u>

Shopping & Ingredients List:

- 8 Prunes
- 50g Cashew Nuts
- 50g Pecan Nuts
- 50g Macadamia Nuts
- 2 tbsp Coconut Oil, melted
- 100g Strawberries, chopped
- 50g Desiccated Coconut, unsweetened

Method

1. In a food processor combine all the ingredients (except the coconut) together until it forms a dough-like mixture. This will take several minutes & will need to use pulse setting intermittently.

2. Using a teaspoon for sizing, take mixture and roll into small truffle like balls.

3. Roll each ball in the coconut. Store in the fridge until required. Can also be frozen.

Nutritional info per serving

Protein	**3.3g**
Carbs	**11.1g**
Fat	**23.4g**
Energy	**268 Kcal**

Super Smoothie (Serves 4)

Shopping & Ingredients List:

- 450g frozen Berries
- 450g light Strawberry Yogurt
- 100ml Skimmed Milk
- 25g Porridge Oats

Method

1. Whizz the berries, yogurt and milk together with a stick blender until smooth. Stir through the porridge oats, then pour into 4 glasses and serve.

Nutritional info per serving

Protein	**8g**
Carbs	**18g**
Fat	**1g**
Energy	**117Kcal**

Here's How To Think Differently And Get Your Body Back

We've all been on a diet and lost weight before. The most challenging part is finding a diet that you can stick to so you can tone up, keep the weight off for good, and fit back into your favourite clothes.

That's where I come in. I help busy ladies like you think differently about your approach to weight loss so you can finally lose the pounds and get your body back..

> **Step 1:** Go to www.**Frucifit.com,** click the "Yes! I Want to Apply for a Free Trial" button and apply for your free trial on my 90-Day Body Transformation Programme.

> **Step 2**: I will get you started on your Body Transformation journey with a bespoke nutrition and exercise strategy. You'll master the basics and use my simple Tone Up system so you don't have to rely on willpower to stop yourself from 'eating your emotions'.

> **Step 3:** You'll receive ongoing support and accountability, and be empowered to take control of your nutrition so you can build a diet to last. We'll closely monitor how you respond and adapt your bespoke plans based on your progress so you can stick to it even on your busiest, most stressful weeks.

Many ladies think they have to give up their favourite foods, spend hours exercising, and go to an intimidating gym to get their body back.

Now you can start to think differently, tone up, and Shift your weight for good.

If you'd like me to help you, go to: www.**Frucifit.com** to get started with your free trial.

Made in the USA
Columbia, SC
02 December 2017